2012)

LIVING WITH DISEASE

HEART

DISEASE

BY LORI DITTMER

CREATIVE EDUCATION

Contents

In 1958, Dr. F. Mason Sones Jr.,

a cardiologist at Cleveland Clinic, discovered that accidents can lead to breakthroughs in medical technology. Sones was about to inject **contrast dye** into a **heart valve** of an awake 26-year-old patient to view the valve on an X-ray. But the **catheter** tip containing the dye accidentally entered the patient's right coronary **artery** instead. Afraid the dye would cause a heart attack, Sones watched as the patient's heart stopped. He shouted for the patient to cough, and the patient's action restarted his heart. Afterward, Sones realized that a smaller amount of dye could be safely injected into the arteries of the heart, allowing physicians to view blockages and diagnose coronary artery disease. The new procedure, known as an angiogram, led to modern heart surgeries such as coronary bypass and angioplasty. It also gave doctors new insight into how heart disease develops and how to slow the progress of the disease in millions of people.

Coronary arteries are vividly displayed with the help of an angiogram.

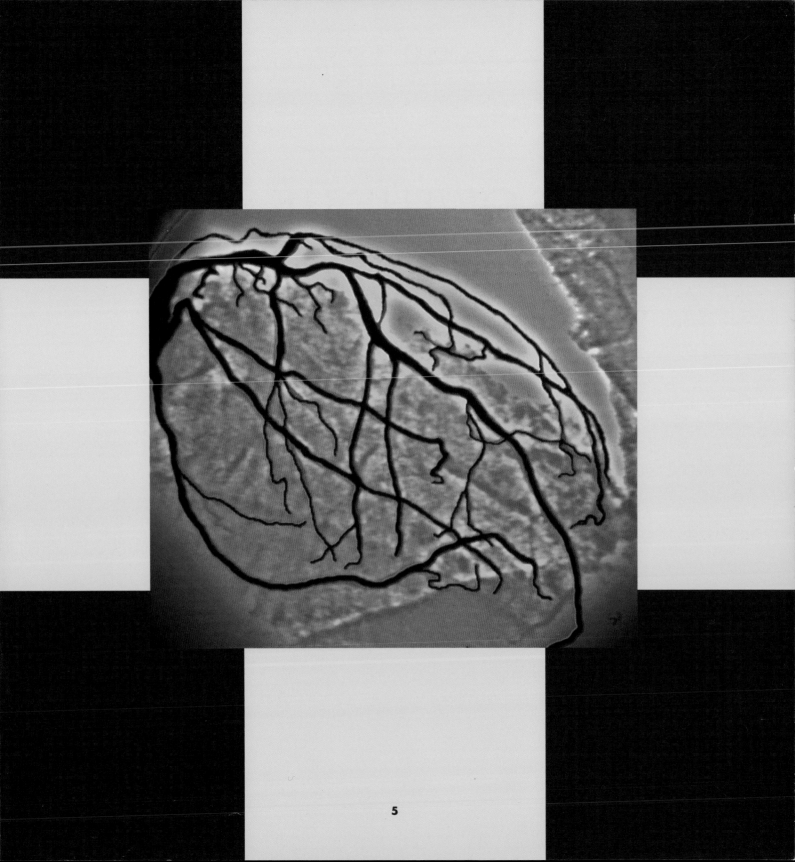

CHAPTER ONE

DISEASES OF THE HEART

The heart, a muscle about the size

of a fist, sits in the middle of the chest, tirelessly pumping blood. But sometimes diseases of the heart prevent the muscle from doing its job. There are many different kinds and causes of heart disease. Most forms are caused by external factors, but some are congenital, which means a person is born with a heart defect, such as a faulty connection between the heart and blood vessels or a heart valve that does not close properly. For every 1,000 live births, 8 or 9 are born with some type of heart defect.

Other people have irregular heartbeats, called arrhythmias, in which the heart rate sporadically speeds up or slows down. Arrhythmias can be congenital, but they can also be caused by a variety of factors, including high blood pressure, heart attack, **rheumatic** heart disease, or certain drugs. Atrial fibrillation, in which the upper chambers of the heart lose their orderly contractions and beat chaotically, is one of the more common arrhythmias, affecting roughly two million Americans.

Sometimes, one type of heart disease causes another. High blood pressure can lead to atherosclerosis, or hardening of the arteries. Both of

The pumping action of the human heart is called the cardiac cycle.

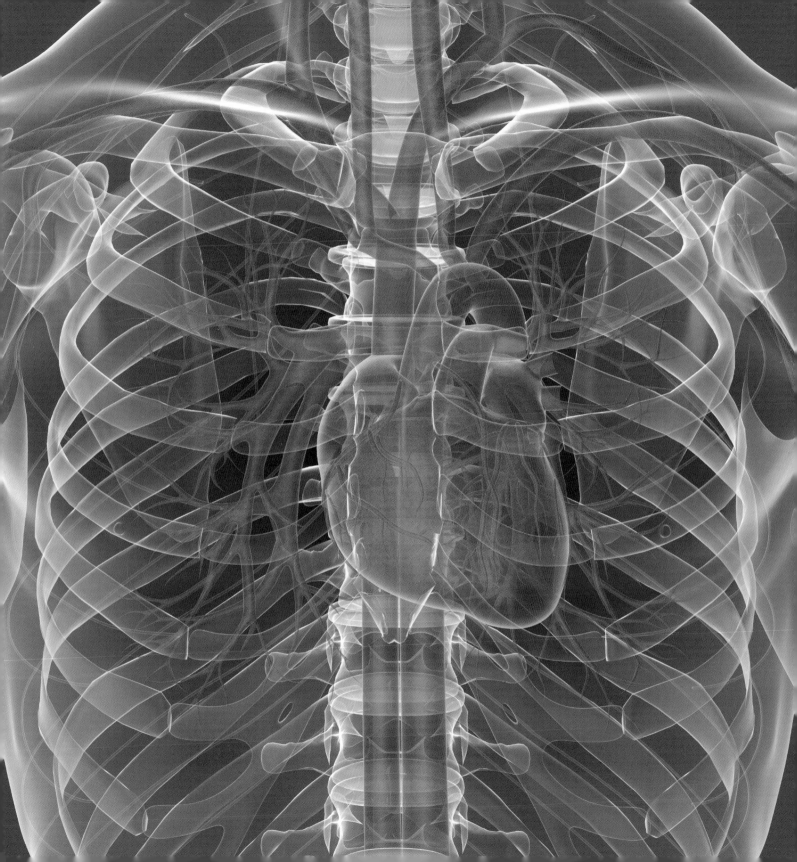

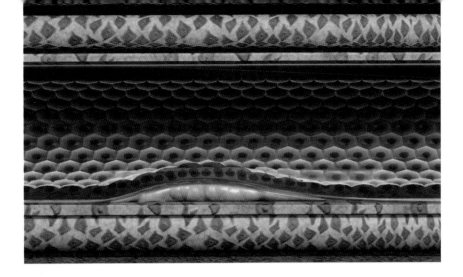

In the above illustration, a buildup of plaque is represented by the yellow area.

these conditions contribute to coronary artery disease, the most common disease of the heart. Coronary artery disease occurs when substances in the blood—including fat, **cholesterol**, and **platelets**—build up as **plaque** on the artery walls and restrict blood flow through the coronary arteries. This condition can cause a heart attack, which can be fatal or lead to a disabling state of heart failure.

Before 1900, people had little experience with heart disease. Many people earned a living performing manual labor, such as farming. Children were also active; they walked to school, performed chores at home, and worked in the fields with their parents. Before automobiles, washing machines, and vacuum cleaners existed, people worked their own gardens, washed clothes by hand, and scrubbed floors and carpets. As the 20th century progressed, however, machines made life easier in **industrialized countries** such as the United States, and they also provided easier access to high-fat foods such as cheese, ice cream, and, eventually, French fries. The combination of less-active lifestyles and rich diets led to more clogged arteries. As a result, heart disease has been the leading cause of death in the U.S. since the early part of the 20th century. Today, it affects more than 12 million Americans and causes 325,000 adult deaths each year.

In recent decades, heart disease has become more prevalent in poorer nations as well, largely because these nations are also becoming more dependent upon machines. According to the World Health Organization (WHO), heart and circulation diseases lead to 30 percent of all deaths worldwide, killing more people than any other cause of death. Roughly 7.2 million people die each year from coronary artery disease.

In general, people who are overweight, exercise very little, or are older than 65 are at higher risk of developing heart disease. Approximately 4 out of 5 people who die from heart disease are 65 or older. Those who have an immediate family member—a parent or a sibling—who has or had heart disease are also more likely to develop it themselves, as some people have **genetic** tendencies toward having high cholesterol or being overweight.

However, these are not the only people who are at risk of developing heart disease. Researchers have discovered that for some people, heart disease begins in childhood. Doctors accidentally stumbled onto the find-

Roughly 75 million American adults have high blood pressure, a type of heart disease that can lead to coronary artery disease. Up to a third of these people do not realize they have high blood pressure because they have no clear symptoms of the condition.

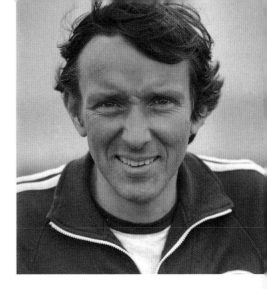

ing while performing **autopsies** on teenaged victims of fatal automobile accidents. Their arteries already showed signs of fatty streaks—the beginning of blocked arteries. In addition, people who are thin, exercise regularly, and have low cholesterol levels can still suffer from heart disease. Jim Fixx, a world-class runner, died suddenly from a heart attack in 1984 at the age of 52. Russian figure skater Sergei Grinkov collapsed on the ice during a practice in 1995. He was 28.

Men are more likely to develop heart disease than women, yet heart disease is the leading cause of death for women in the U.S. and Canada. During their younger years, women receive some protection against heart disease from the **hormone** estrogen. As they age, they lose this protection, and a woman's risk for heart disease at age 55 becomes similar to a man's risk at age 45. More than 350,000 American women die from coronary artery disease each year.

Symptoms of heart disease include shortness of breath, periodic pain, pressure in the chest, fatigue, or heart **palpitations**. Chest pain or pressure, known as angina, is the symptom most often associated with heart disease. Angina is not a heart attack, and it usually does not cause permanent damage to the heart. However, angina is the body's warning that something is

Jim Fixx began running when he was in his mid-30s to lose weight.

A President's Quadruple Bypass

In September 2004, fewer than four years after leaving the White House, former U.S. president Bill Clinton entered the hospital complaining of chest pain and shortness of breath. He was 58 years old at the time. Although Clinton—who was known for eating fast food throughout his presidency—had no history of heart problems, he did have high cholesterol. During his four-hour quadruple bypass, the surgeon rerouted four coronary arteries. Some of the arteries were 90 percent blocked. If Clinton had not had the surgery when he did, he almost certainly would have suffered a major heart attack within a few months. After his close call, Clinton joined the American Heart Association to launch a campaign encouraging kids to eat healthier and to exercise. In 2010, Clinton had an angioplasty on one of the same arteries that had been bypassed nearly six years earlier but had become blocked again.

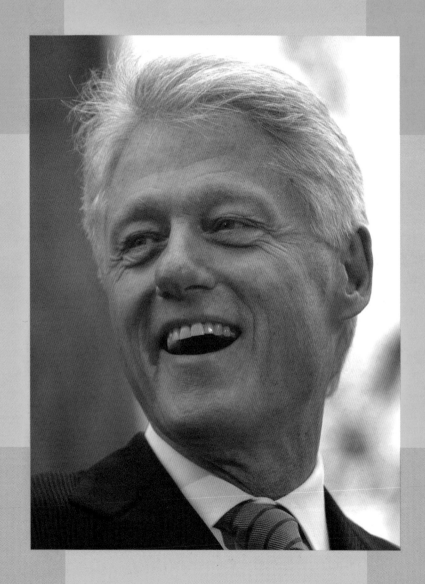

A few weeks after
his 2004 surgery,
Bill Clinton was back
on his feet.

wrong. A person who experiences angina should contact a physician right away to make a treatment plan that may prevent a heart attack.

Although many people with heart disease experience angina, researchers estimate that 3 to 4 million Americans have silent ischemia, characterized by an unnoticed but persistent decreased blood flow to the heart. The body's usual warning system — chest pain — fails to register, so in such cases, a fatal heart attack might be the first and only sign of this form of heart disease. Roughly half of all heart disease deaths are sudden and unexpected.

The most dangerous outcome of coronary artery disease is a heart attack, which occurs when blood cannot flow to a part of the heart muscle. Symptoms include uncomfortable pressure or tightness in the chest, pain that lasts more than 30 minutes, light-headedness, nausea, shortness of breath, and pain that spreads to the shoulders, neck, or arms. Women's symptoms sometimes differ from men's. While a man may initially feel chest pressure or pain, a woman might feel back pain or nausea.

People who think they might be having a heart attack need immediate medical help. A common, often fatal, mistake is to blame heart attack symptoms on stress or indigestion. The longer the heart goes without blood, the more damaged it becomes.

BY THE NUMBERS **Timing is critical when it comes to saving a person who might be having a heart attack. More than 70,000 Canadians and 1.5 million Americans suffer a heart attack each year. About half of them die. Of those who die, 50 percent die within the first hour, before they even seek medical help.**

CHAPTER TWO

HEARTS UNDER ATTACK

The heart is divided into four parts,

or chambers. The right and left ventricles make up the lower chambers of the heart, while the right and left atria (plural for "atrium") are at the top. These chambers contract to squeeze blood out and then relax and expand to let more blood flow in. Imagine holding a soft plastic bottle underwater. When you squeeze, the water squirts out, and when you release your grip, the bottle sucks more water back in.

The right side of the heart pumps blood through the lungs. There, the blood picks up oxygen and gets rid of carbon dioxide. The left side of the heart takes the oxygen-filled blood and pumps it out the aorta, the body's largest artery. Other major arteries branch off from the aorta and transport blood through smaller blood vessels, which in turn carry blood throughout the body. The coronary arteries, which come out of the aorta, surround the surface of the heart, providing it with its own supply of blood. The coronary arteries must be strong and **elastic** to handle changes in blood flow when the heart needs more oxygen, particularly during exercise. But, over the course of many years, the arteries can become damaged, even diseased.

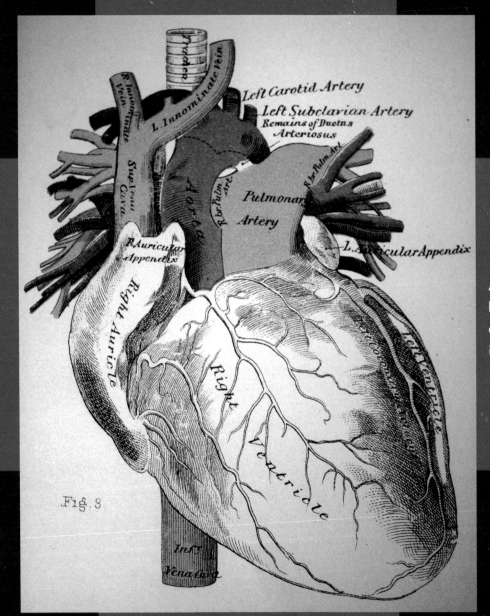

Left Carotid Artery
Left Subclavian Artery
Remains of Ductus
Arteriosus

L. Innominate Vein
R. Innominate Vein
Trachea
Sup. Vena Cava
Aorta
R. br. Pulm. Art.
Pulmonary Artery
R. br. Pulm. Art.
L. Auricular Appendix
R. Auricular Appendix
Right Auricle
Right Ventricle
Left Ventricle
Fig. 3
Inf. Vena Cava

An illustration of a
heart from a medical
dictionary printed
in 1882.

HEARTS UNDER ATTACK

The main culprit behind coronary artery disease is atherosclerosis. In the past, researchers compared blood vessels to a system of pipes. When dirt and other materials stick to the sides of a pipe, less water can flow through it. In the same way, as plaque accumulates in the coronary arteries, less blood can flow through them to reach the heart.

In the late 1980s and early 1990s, researchers began using ultrasound technology (which produces sound waves directed into the body to create an image of structures beneath the skin) to get a clear interior view of coronary arteries. Ultrasounds can detect differences between solids and fluids, and researchers were able to confirm that, in some cases, plaque does clog arteries, as in the pipe illustration explained above, leading to a heart attack. They also found that even though an artery might appear to be clear of plaque, buildup can take place within the wall of an artery, accumulating outward without narrowing the artery. This hardens the artery, which decreases its flexibility. If the arteries cannot expand to allow more blood to flow when the heart needs it, the heart does not receive enough oxygen.

Many physicians believe that the smaller, less noticeable plaques that build up within the artery walls can be more dangerous than visible plaques because they are more likely to be unstable and to rupture,

Framingham Heart Study

In 1948, the National Heart Institute (now called the National Heart, Lung and Blood Institute) enrolled 5,209 people from Framingham, Massachusetts, in an observational study. After years of watching these men and women, who were all between the ages of 30 and 62 at the beginning of the study, researchers learned a great deal about heart disease. They began to understand the risk factors for heart disease and realized that some—such as smoking, high cholesterol, and a less-active lifestyle—were within a person's control. Before the study, doctors believed that high blood pressure was supposed to increase as people age. In 1971, the study enrolled 5,124 more participants—the adult children of the original group and their spouses. Today, the study includes the grandchildren of the original members. Since the beginning of the study, more than 1,000 scientific papers have been written about the Framingham data.

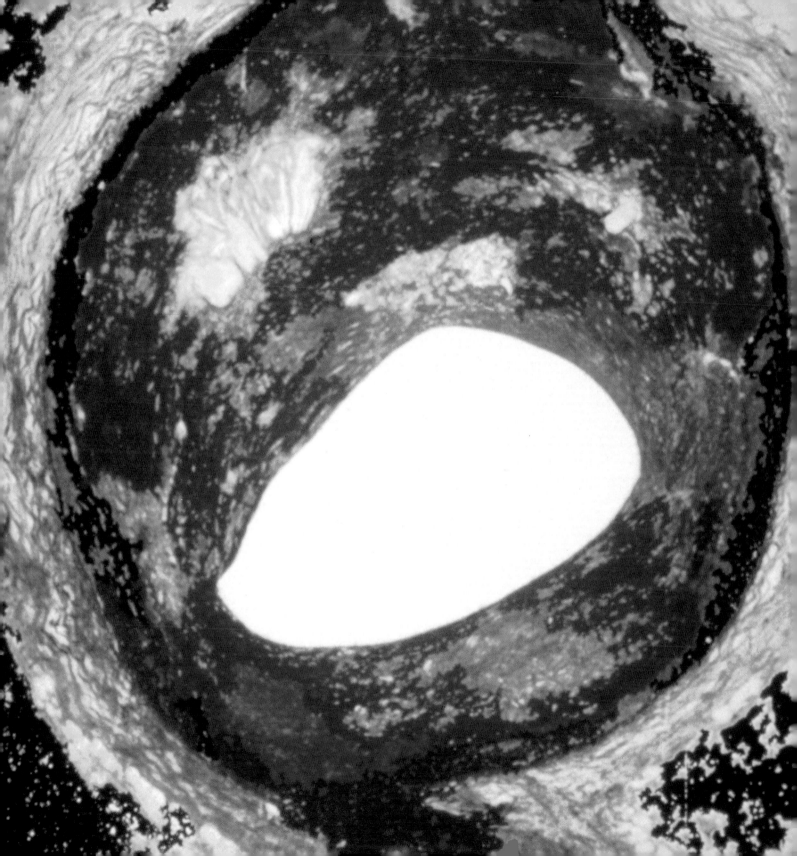

leaving a crack in the plaque. The body thinks the rupture is an injury in the artery wall and creates a blood **clot** at that site to repair it. The clot might decrease blood flow enough to cause angina or a heart attack.

If blood flow is blocked for longer than 30 minutes, part of the heart muscle will become damaged or die. Unlike angina, the damage from a heart attack is permanent. The amount of injury to the heart depends on the size of the area deprived of blood and the time it takes for the patient to receive treatment to restore blood flow. When the heart heals, it forms scar tissue, which does not contract or pump as well as healthy tissue. Even 10 percent damage to the heart impairs its functioning. When 25 percent of the heart muscle is harmed, the heart becomes enlarged and cannot pump as much blood with as much force as it did before. This is called heart failure. Because the heart loses pumping power, some of the blood pools in veins, arteries, lungs, and other organs. This can cause shortness of breath and swelling in the legs, stomach, and liver. As the damage to the heart reaches 40 percent, the person will likely go into **shock** or die.

A heart attack can cause complications such as recurrent chest pain, arrhythmias, or pericarditis, which is an inflammation of the pericardium, the outer lining of the heart. Heart attacks can also cause more

When an artery is clogged by plaque (red-orange in the image at left), blood cannot flow properly through it.

urgent conditions. When the lower chambers of the heart beat chaotically, the ventricles cannot pump enough blood to the rest of the body. Without immediate treatment, the patient will lose consciousness or die from this condition, called ventricular fibrillation.

Medical experts believe that several factors work together to bring about the plaque-lined arteries that can lead to a heart attack. Some risk factors—including sex, age, and family history—are beyond a person's control. But other risk factors are within one's power to change. These factors include high cholesterol, high blood pressure, and smoking. Having more than one risk factor multiplies a person's risk for developing coronary artery disease.

Everyone has cholesterol. The liver makes most of the cholesterol a person needs. Extra cholesterol comes from food, such as meat, egg yolks, and dairy products. There are two kinds of cholesterol: low-density lipoprotein (LDL) is the "bad" cholesterol, and high-density lipoprotein (HDL) is the "good" one. Too much LDL cholesterol in the blood can build up in coronary arteries.

Blood pressure is a measurement of the force of the blood on the artery walls. Normal blood pressure is 120/80 or lower. The top number reflects the pressure on the walls

Because cholesterol is a soft, fatty substance, it cannot dissolve in the bloodstream.

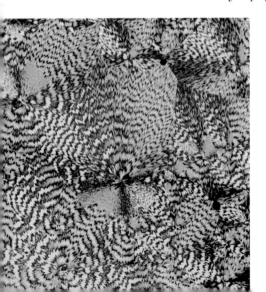

More than 1 billion adults worldwide are overweight, and 300 million are obese. Carrying extra weight increases a person's risk for high blood pressure, high cholesterol, and other heart diseases. Obesity levels around the globe range from 5 percent in China and Japan to 75 percent in the South Pacific islands of Samoa.

Smoking causes 20 percent of all deaths due to heart disease. In addition, a smoker is twice as likely as a nonsmoker to suffer from a heart attack. After about 10 years of not smoking, however, a former smoker's risk of having a heart attack is nearly as low as a nonsmoker's.

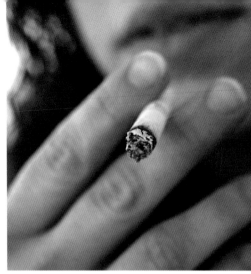

as the heart contracts; the bottom number shows the pressure on the walls when the heart is relaxed. When blood pressure climbs above normal levels, it means that the heart is working harder than normal to keep blood flowing. When blood pressure remains high for a long time, the blood vessels become tighter and narrower, and the heart, like any other muscle with an increased workload, grows larger and thicker. When the heart can no longer adapt to the large workload, it weakens and loses its pumping efficiency.

Smoking increases the risk of heart disease because tobacco smoke contains many substances, such as the toxic chemicals in tar and nicotine, which raise blood pressure and heart rate, cause arteries to narrow, make blood more likely to clot, increase LDL cholesterol, and lower HDL cholesterol. Smoking also irritates the inner lining of the artery walls, making them more likely to attract plaque buildup.

A smoker has a greater risk of developing heart disease over lung cancer.

CHAPTER THREE

LINES OF DEFENSE

To arrive at a diagnosis of coronary artery disease, a cardiologist will look at a patient's medical and family history and other risk factors. The doctor will perform a variety of tests, including a blood test to check for fat and cholesterol levels. He or she will also order a chest X-ray to look for existing heart failure and take another type of X-ray called a coronary angiogram to view the coronary arteries.

When coronary arteries are so narrowed by blockages that they almost disappear on an angiogram, doctors take action.

There is no cure for heart disease. Someone diagnosed with the disease must make lifestyle and behavior changes to lessen the risk of heart attack or other complications. The first line of defense against coronary artery disease involves eating a heart-healthy, low-fat diet. People who reduce their total and LDL cholesterol levels by 10 to 15 percent reduce their heart disease risk by up to 30 percent. The typical **Western** diet is composed of 35 to 45 percent fat, which health experts agree is too high. Doctors recommend that less than 30 percent of a person's diet come from fat.

Regular exercise is also an important part of fighting heart disease. Exercise lowers blood pressure and LDL cholesterol and helps prevent

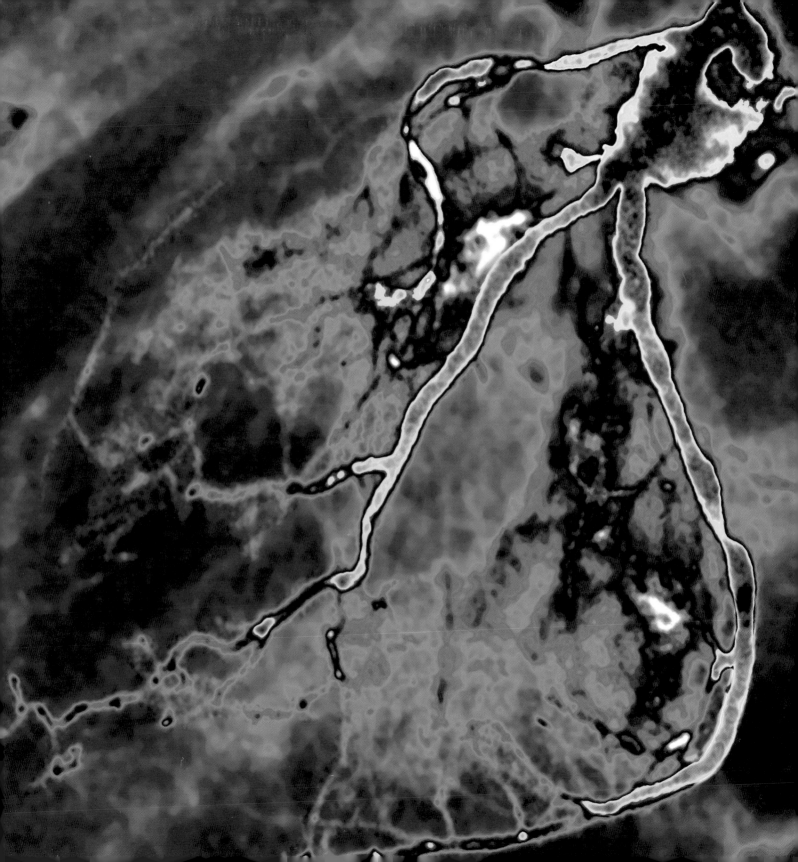

blood clots. Taking a 30-minute walk every day can reduce a person's risk of having a heart attack by almost 50 percent. Even people who have already had a heart attack can benefit from starting an exercise program under their doctor's supervision. Exercise can lower the risk of a second heart attack by up to 60 percent.

Smokers can help to prevent or delay heart disease by quitting. Even people who have smoked for 30 or 40 years can benefit from quitting. Smokers who have already had a heart attack and then quit smoking reduce their risk for a second heart attack by 50 percent.

Sometimes lifestyle changes are not enough to decrease the risk of a heart attack. Doctors commonly prescribe medications to help people control their heart disease. But taking medicine does not excuse people from also having to work hard to change unhealthy habits. The best results happen when medicine, diet, exercise, and other healthy choices work together.

For patients with high blood pressure or narrowed arteries, doctors might prescribe anti-anginal drugs called beta blockers. Taken regularly, these drugs decrease heart rate and lessen the force of the heart's beating. This keeps the heart from becoming overworked and damaged. Nitrates, which patients take prior to physical activity, help

Experts recommend that people keep their total cholesterol level below 200 milligrams per deciliter of blood (mg/dl). More than half of Americans' cholesterol levels are higher than that. Once a person's cholesterol reaches 300 mg/dl, his or her risk of dying from coronary artery disease is 4 times greater than someone with a cholesterol level of 150 mg/dl.

An Unforeseen Heart Attack

Tim Russert, a television news personality and moderator of the talk show *Meet the Press*, collapsed from a massive heart attack at his desk on June 13, 2008. Emergency workers arrived just three minutes after receiving the 911 call, but they were unable to revive him. Before his heart attack, Russert, 58, had been diagnosed with coronary artery disease. Doctors said his condition was "asymptomatic," meaning that he did not feel pain from his narrowed blood vessels. Russert was taking medication and exercising to control the disease, which made the sudden heart attack more surprising. Russert's doctor later explained that a piece of cholesterol likely broke free from an artery wall and lodged itself in a vessel, blocking blood flow to Russert's left ventricle. When the heart attack deprived Russert's heart of blood, it went into ventricular fibrillation and began to quiver, unable to pump blood properly to Russert's body or brain.

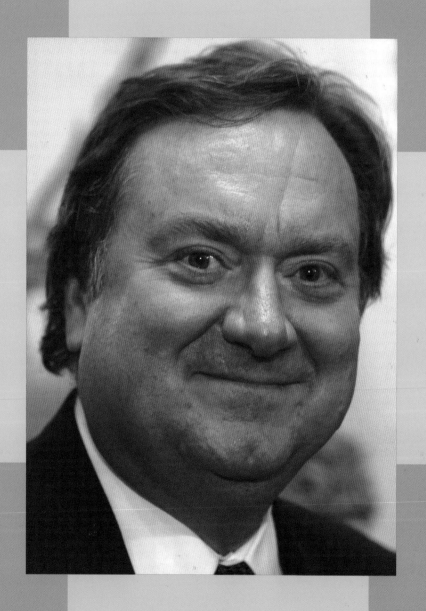

Tim Russert spent most of his adult life involved with politics and broadcast journalism.

to relieve angina by temporarily widening the coronary arteries. People who have heart disease as a result of high cholesterol sometimes take drugs called statins, which block a substance the liver uses to make cholesterol. These drugs can help to reduce LDL levels by up to 40 percent.

Doctors sometimes prescribe blood thinners, such as warfarin, to keep clots from forming in the arteries. Although it's not a prescription drug, aspirin is also a blood thinner. With a doctor's approval, it can be taken by people who have already had a heart attack or stroke to improve blood flow through blocked arteries.

In some cases, lifestyle changes and medication cannot do enough to reduce artery blockages. Some people must have surgery to reopen or reroute clogged vessels. Physicians generally perform either angioplasty or bypass surgery on patients with severely blocked arteries.

During an angioplasty, the cardiologist makes an **incision** in a patient's upper thigh. Then a long, thin tube called a balloon-tipped guide catheter is fed through the artery in the leg to the site of the blockage. The doctor watches the progress of the guide catheter through X-ray images on a TV monitor. Once the catheter is positioned in the blockage, the doctor inflates the balloon. This pushes the plaque against the artery wall, widening the artery and allowing more blood to flow

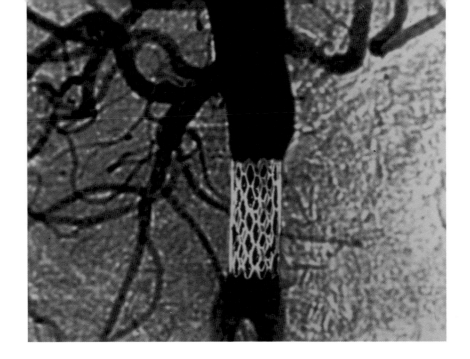

through. Usually, a stent—a tiny mesh tube—is wrapped around the deflated balloon tip and attaches to the artery wall when the balloon inflates. The stent remains in the body to prop the artery open.

In patients with severe artery blockage, doctors often turn to coronary artery bypass graft (CABG) surgery. The surgery does just what it says: doctors "bypass" a clogged artery with part of a blood vessel taken from the chest or leg. A vein from the leg is stitched to the aorta and connected to the affected artery, whereas a vein from the chest is stitched directly to the diseased coronary artery. One end of the "new" vein is attached above the blockage and the other below it, allowing blood to loop around the blockage and flow to the heart. As many as four blocked arteries can be dealt with in one CABG surgery. This surgery improves symptoms in 85 percent of patients. However, in 40 percent of

Doctors closely monitor the progress of a stent being inserted through a guide catheter.

At rest, the heart of an average healthy adult pumps three ounces (89 ml) of blood with each beat. The blood travels through the body and back to the heart in about one minute. Over the course of a day, this work amounts to more than 2,000 gallons (7,571 l) of blood flowing through the heart.

bypass patients, blockages can recur in the new arteries or in previously unblocked arteries within about 10 years.

Sometimes a patient's heart disease is so extreme that it leads to a heart attack. The most important step in treating a heart attack is to restore blood flow to the heart before any part of the muscle dies. Medications that dissolve blood clots are commonly given within the first two hours of the beginning of a heart attack. One study showed that 75 percent of patients who were treated with clot-dissolving drugs within the first 70 minutes of the start of heart attack symptoms survived with little or no heart damage. After six hours, much of the damage is already done, and it is too late for clot-dissolving drugs.

Doctors also often give heart attack patients drugs to widen blood vessels or to decrease the workload of the heart. They might perform an emergency angioplasty to clear the artery blockage. If the heart attack causes an irregular heartbeat, the doctor will administer drugs or use an external defibrillator, an electric device that jolts the heart back into its normal rhythm. Patients who are still alive two hours after the start of a heart attack are likely to survive, but they might have complications. Within a few days, many patients undergo an angioplasty or CABG surgery to help prevent a second heart attack.

CHAPTER FOUR

REPAIR AND RENEWAL

Technology has made incredible gains

over the last century; 100 years ago, the only way for physicians to clearly see what was happening in the coronary arteries was to examine them after someone had died. Many researchers tested their theories and new tools on themselves. German doctor Werner Forssmann inserted the first documented human cardiac catheter into his own body in 1929. He was testing a theory that drugs for cardiac **resuscitation** could be administered directly to the heart. Forssmann inserted the catheter into the vein at the base of the elbow and directed it toward his heart. He then walked to another part of the hospital to have an X-ray taken, which showed the catheter resting in his right atrium.

Since then, knowledge of coronary artery disease has grown by leaps and bounds. In the 1980s, doctors began using intravascular ultrasound—by which a special catheter featuring an ultrasound probe is threaded into a coronary artery—to view cross-sections of artery walls. This enabled doctors to more accurately measure plaque levels and determine the best course of action.

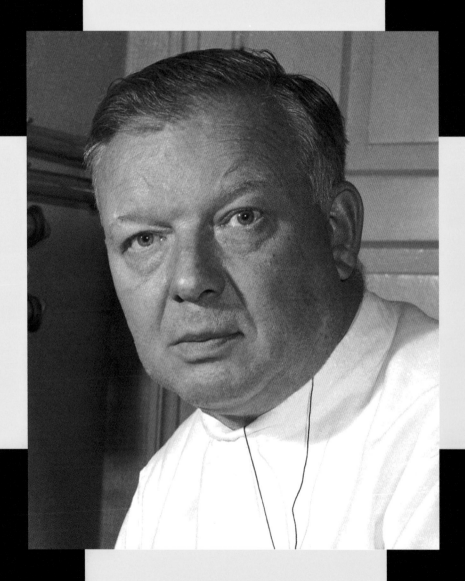

Werner Forssmann shared the 1956 Nobel Prize in Physiology or Medicine with the two doctors who put his catheterization into practice.

Every 34 seconds, someone in the U.S. suffers a heart attack. Each year, about 785,000 Americans experience a heart attack for the first time, while 470,000 have a recurrent attack. In addition, an estimated 10 million Americans suffer from angina.

While angioplasty and CABG surgery are the main procedures used on blocked arteries today, doctors continue to research and develop new methods. For a traditional CABG surgery, a surgeon must make an incision over the sternum, or breastbone, and split the bone to get to the patient's heart. During the surgery, the heart does not beat, so the patient is put on a heart-lung machine, which pumps oxygenated blood through the body. A newer procedure, the off-pump coronary artery bypass (OPCAB), calls for the surgeon to work on the heart while it is beating. Early studies have shown that OPCAB surgeries result in fewer complications, such as stroke, memory loss, or bleeding.

For patients who need treatment for only one or two arteries, surgeons can perform another off-pump procedure known as a minimally **invasive** direct coronary artery bypass (MIDCAB). This employs a smaller incision site between the ribs and does not require the breaking of the sternum. As a result, MIDCAB causes less bleeding, lowers the risk of infection, and ensures a faster and less painful recovery time for the patient.

An even less invasive procedure is robotically assisted heart surgery, in which the surgeon drills three dime-sized holes, called ports, in the chest. A tiny video camera and surgical instruments attached to

The Evolution of Bypass Surgery

Today, coronary artery bypass grafting is a fairly common procedure. Doctors perform the surgery on about 500,000 patients in the U.S. every year. Only 60 years ago, though, researchers were just figuring out how the procedure might work. During the 1940s and '50s, surgeons performed open-heart surgery on animals. The doctors cooled the animals' hearts to the level of hypothermia (a core body temperature lower than 95 °F, or 35 °C) to slow the heart's pumping enough to operate on small arteries and veins. In the 1950s, the development of the heart-lung machine, which keeps blood circulating while the heart is stopped during surgery, helped protect patients undergoing heart procedures. Argentine doctor René Favaloro, a surgeon at the Cleveland Clinic, performed the first documented CABG surgery in 1967. Within a year, 171 bypass surgeries had been performed at the clinic.

robotic arms are inserted through the holes, and the surgeon operates by watching a video monitor and controlling the robotic system with a computer. The small ports allow these patients to heal faster, leave the hospital sooner, and recover much more quickly than patients of other bypass surgeries. One disadvantage of this procedure is its cost; it can top $1 million for a hospital to purchase the system, not counting yearly maintenance fees.

Someday, patients might be able to have their coronary arteries repaired or replaced without ever having surgery. Scientists are currently studying the therapeutic potential of angiogenesis, the process of growing new blood vessels from existing ones. Everyone has collateral vessels, or tiny arteries that are normally closed. Sometimes, when a blockage forms in the coronary arteries or in the brain's blood vessels, collateral vessels open and connect larger arteries or parts of the same artery, helping to re-route oxygen-rich blood around blocked areas. Angiogenesis naturally takes place within some bodies to grow new collateral vessels.

Researchers do not know why angiogenesis occurs in some people and not others, though. They have found that certain substances, called growth factors, help trigger new blood vessel growth. Using gene therapy, doctors could administer these growth factors to the hearts of patients with severely blocked arteries. Clinical studies have suggested that patients receiving gene therapy report having less angina. Gene therapy also appeared to prevent re-stenosis, or the recurrence of artery blockage after a patient has undergone traditional heart surgery. However, no angiogenic drug had been approved for use in the U.S. as of 2011.

Another non-surgical treatment for heart disease might be found in stem cells. While most cells cannot change (for example, a skin cell cannot become a blood cell), stem cells can become any kind of cell anywhere in the body. Introducing stem cells into a sickly portion of the body could possibly stimulate a recovery as the healthy cells multiply and take over for sick ones. Most stem cells used in research and treatments are adult stem cells (which are found in both children and adults). These cells commonly originate in **bone marrow** or the blood from an umbilical cord that connects a mother and baby until birth. However, the use of stem cells is a **controversial** area of research because other stem cells can come from **embryos** that have been scheduled to be discarded by fertility clinics. Harvesting embryonic stem cells has raised moral and ethical questions that researchers, patients, and the general public continue to debate.

Embryonic stem cells used in research are taken from eggs that have been fertilized in a lab dish or test tube.

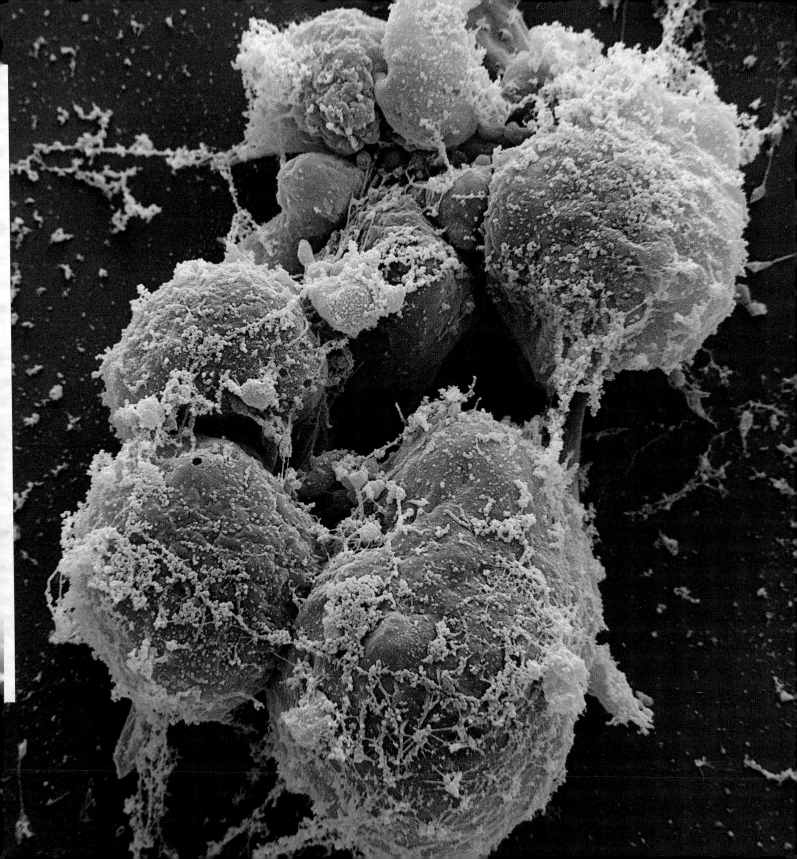

In 2001, researchers began testing the use of stem cells on mice and rats whose hearts had been damaged by heart attack. After injecting adult bone marrow cells into the walls of the damaged mouse hearts, they found that the stem cells transformed into heart muscle cells, developing a new network of arteries to feed the heart—a result that suggests the procedure has the potential to restore a damaged heart's function and pumping power.

The WHO predicts that in the future, heart disease patients will wear tiny computers that can record their health information, screening for early signs of heart problems. Furthermore, instead of a human physician performing surgery, "nano-surgeons"—miniscule robots capable of scraping away plaque, repairing damaged artery walls, and delivering drugs to hard-to-reach areas near the heart—might be sent into the arteries.

Within the past century, scientists have made great strides in understanding heart disease. Although there might never be a cure for coronary artery disease, doctors have gained new insights into preventing the disease, slowing its progression, and treating it. That work has meant longer, healthier lives for millions of people.

An adult weighing 150 pounds (68 kg) has roughly 5 quarts (4.7 l) of blood. If his or her blood vessels were laid end to end, they'd cover about 100,000 miles (160,934 km)— long enough to circle the Earth nearly 4 times at the equator.

GLOSSARY

artery: a blood vessel, or tube, that carries blood away from the heart to other parts of the body

autopsies: examinations of a body's vital organs after death to determine the cause of death

bone marrow: the tissue within bones where blood cells are created

catheter: a hollow, flexible tube inserted into a body channel, such as an artery, to allow the passage of fluids

cholesterol: a soft, waxy substance found in the bloodstream and all cells that is used to help digest fats and strengthen cell membranes; it can cause heart problems when it builds up in the blood

clot: a thick or solid mass or lump formed from a liquid, such as blood

contrast dye: a substance used in an X-ray to get a better view of images within the body

controversial: causing a dispute between two sides with opposing views

elastic: flexible and stretchable

embryos: human offspring in the early stages of development, from the time an egg is fertilized until the eighth week

genetic: having to do with the genes, the basic units of instruction in a cell, which control a person's physical traits and pass characteristics from parents to offspring

heart valve: a valve that controls the one-way flow of blood to or from the heart

hormone: a substance produced by the body that affects activity within the body, such as growth

incision: a cut performed during surgery

industrialized countries: nations that have developed industries on a wide scale

invasive: involving entering the body by puncture or incision during a medical procedure

obese: having a body weight more than 20 percent greater than recommended for a specific height

palpitations: noticeably fast, strong, or irregular heartbeats

plaque: a fatty deposit made up of cholesterol and other substances that collects on or within artery walls

platelets: disk-shaped cells in the blood that promote clotting

resuscitation: the act of reviving or bringing back to consciousness or life

rheumatic: relating to or caused by rheumatism, or inflammation or pain in the muscles and joints; rheumatic heart disease is brought on by rheumatic fever

shock: a medical condition involving very low blood pressure, confusion, poor breathing, and clammy skin, which can result from blood loss, heart failure, or other bodily trauma

Western: having to do with the western part of the world, particularly Europe and North America

BIBLIOGRAPHY

Cohen, Barry M., and Bobbie Hasselbring. *Coronary Heart Disease: A Guide to Diagnosis and Treatment.* 2nd ed. Omaha, Neb.: Addicus Books, 2007.

Gersh, Bernard, ed. *Mayo Clinic Heart Book: The Ultimate Guide to Heart Health.* New York: William Morrow and Company, 2000.

Lipsky, Martin, Marla Mendelson, Stephen Havas, and Michael Miller. *American Medical Association Guide to Preventing and Treating Heart Disease: Essential Information You and Your Family Need to Know about Having a Healthy Heart.* Hoboken, N.J.: John Wiley & Sons, 2008.

Mackay, Judith, and George Mensah. "The Atlas of Heart Disease and Stroke." World Health Organization. http://www.who.int/cardiovascular_diseases/ resources/atlas/en.

Mehta, Nirav J., and Ijaz A. Khan. "Cardiology's 10 Greatest Discoveries of the 20th Century." *Texas Heart Institute Journal* 29 no. 3. (2002): 164–171.

Nordqvist, Christian. "Bill Clinton to Undergo Heart Surgery Again Today." *Medical News Today*, March 10, 2005.

Rimmerman, Curtis Mark. *Heart Attack: A Cleveland Clinic Guide.* Cleveland, Ohio: Cleveland Clinic Press, 2006.

Sternberg, Steve. "Russert Death Shows Heart Attack Isn't Easy to Predict." *USA Today*, June 16, 2008.

FURTHER READING

Hurst, J. Willis. *The Heart: The Kids' Questions and Answer Book.* New York: McGraw-Hill, 1999.

Sheen, Barbara. *Heart Disease.* Farmington Hills, Mich.: Lucent Books, 2004.

Wiese, Jim. *Head to Toe Science: Over 40 Eye-Popping, Spine-Tingling, Heart-Pounding Activities That Teach Kids about the Human Body.* New York: John Wiley & Sons, 2000.

Stoyles, Pennie. *The A–Z of Health.* Vol. 3, F–J. North Mankato, Minn.: Smart Apple Media, 2011.

INDEX

Published by Creative Education • P.O. Box 227, Mankato, Minnesota 56002
Creative Education is an imprint of The Creative Company
www.thecreativecompany.us
Design and production by The Design Lab • Art direction by Rita Marshall
Printed by Corporate Graphics in the United States of America
Photographs by Alamy (Phototake Inc.), AP Images (Jerry Mosey, Kathy Willens), Corbis (Bettmann,
David Scharf/Science Faction), Getty Images (3DClinic, CMSP, David Malin, Justin Sullivan,
ZEPHYR/SPL), iStockphoto (Trent Chambers, Sebastian Kaulitzki, Mark Strozier)
Copyright © 2012 Creative Education
International copyright reserved in all countries. No part of this book may be reproduced in any
form without written permission from the publisher.
Library of Congress Cataloging-in-Publication Data
Dittmer, Lori. Heart disease / by Lori Dittmer. p. cm. — (Living with disease)
Includes bibliographical references and index. Summary: A look at heart disease, examining the
ways in which it develops, its symptoms and diagnosis, the effects it has on a person's daily life,
and improvements in medicinal and surgical treatments.
ISBN 978-1-60818-075-2
1. Heart—Diseases—Juvenile literature. I. Title.
RC673.D58 2011   616.1'2—dc22   2010030365

CPSIA: 110310 PO1384
First Edition 9 8 7 6 5 4 3 2 1